Adult Safeguarding

SHARING GOOD PRACTICE SERIES

Adult Safeguarding

Could We Do Better?
A Trainer's Perspective

A Guide for all Social and Health Care Staff,
Students, Family, Friends and the General Public

Bob Dawson RMN, RNLD

THE CHOIR PRESS

Copyright © 2021 Bob Dawson

All rights reserved. No part of this publication may be reproduced or transmitted in any form or by any means, electronic or mechanical including photocopying, recording or any information storage or retrieval system, without prior permission in writing from the publishers.

The right of Bob Dawson to be identified as the author of this work has been asserted by him in accordance with the Copyright, Designs and Patents Act 1988

First published in the United Kingdom in 2021 by
The Choir Press

ISBN 978-1-78963-238-5

Disclaimer.

The publisher and the author are providing this book and its contents on an "as is" basis and make no representations or warranties of any kind with respect to this book or its contents. The publisher and the author disclaim all such representations and warranties, including but not limited to warranties of healthcare for a particular purpose. In addition, the publisher and the author assume no responsibility for errors, inaccuracies, omissions, or any other inconsistencies herein.

The content of this book is for informational purposes only and is not intended to diagnose, treat, cure, or prevent any condition or disease. You understand that this book is not intended as a substitute for consultation with a qualified medical practitioner. Please consult with your own physician or healthcare specialist regarding the suggestions and recommendations made in this book. The use of this book implies your acceptance of this disclaimer.

The publisher and the author make no guarantees concerning the level of success you may experience by following the advice and strategies contained in this book, and you accept the risk that results will differ for each individual.

Contents

Foreword ix

Introduction xi

1. What is the difference between safeguarding procedures and good practice? 2
2. What happened before *No Secrets* 1999? 3
3. What has changed since *No Secrets* was implemented? 5
4. Who does safeguarding affect? 6
5. What was the impact of *Making Safeguarding Personal* 2014? 7
6. What has changed since the Care Act 2014 was implemented? 9
7. What are the six key principles of the Care Act 2014? 11
8. What are the different categories of abuse? 12
9. Who can abuse? 14
10. What might you witness, hear or discover that you need to take further? 17
11. What systems in place where you work are aimed at reducing the risk of abuse occurring? 19
12. Why may some staff and others not report suspected abuse? 22
13. Six-step exercise for managers and staff teams to enhance good practice. 24
14. What is the role of the safeguarding adult's board? 33
15. What is the role of the local authority safeguarding team? 35
16. Should I raise a concern, relative/member of the public? 36
17. Where does confidentiality/information sharing fit in? 37

18.	What is the duty of candour?	38
19.	What do I do if I feel the abuse is not deliberate?	38
20.	What if the person allegedly being abused does not want us to raise a concern?	40
21.	What should I expect if I raise a concern?	41
22.	What can I do if I am unhappy with how a safeguarding concern is being dealt with?	42
23.	What is the role of the service manager in safeguarding?	43
24.	As a service manager what support should I expect from my superiors?	46
25.	What is a section 42 enquiry (commonly know as a safeguarding enquiry)?	47
26.	Whose policy should we follow?	48
27.	What is the value of training in this area?	48
28.	What is the role of the Care Quality Commission?	51
29.	What is the difference between individual and organisational abuse?	52
30.	How are organisational abuse enquiries carried out?	55
31.	How are staff protected by safeguarding?	57
32.	What is the impact of abuse?	59

Appendix 1 Early Indicators of Concern in Care Services (Organisational Abuse) 61

Appendix 2 Useful website addresses 71

Acknowledgements

To Dee for proof reading, multiple ideas to improve the text and for always being there. As this is an area both of us have been actively involved in since 1999 her input was invaluable.

To Judy for writing the foreword, proof reading and for the years we trained together. Almost all her suggestions coming from the proof reading are now part of the text.

To all the participants of all the training sessions, over many years, a number of the comments which have found their way into the text are yours.

To the staff at the Choir Press. Miles, Rachel, Adrian and Josh, you make a process which could be anxiety provoking a real pleasure. Always cheerful, patient, and full of helpful ideas and responses. You all made this process enjoyable and fulfilling for me, thank you.

Foreword

Although the concept of adult safeguarding has been in existence since the publication of *No Secrets* in 2000, it still causes many service providers anxiety – a fear that they will be blamed or criticised when things go wrong, and not given the opportunity to put things right. This book gives those services who work with adults who have care and support needs, and who are risk of abuse or neglect, the opportunity to think about adult safeguarding in a more positive light.

Adult safeguarding is not just reacting after someone has been abused or neglected. It is about thinking about things before they happen and planning to try to prevent things from going wrong in the first place. It is about giving people the skills and the confidence to speak up when they think something is not right, and to work in partnership with others to stop things getting worse.

This book encourages people to talk about adult safeguarding and to accept it as a fundamental part of working with adults who have care and support needs. Most importantly it helps us to acknowledge that we all have a part to play in keeping the people we care for safe from abuse.

Judy Eke
Adult Safeguarding Manager
South Gloucestershire Council

Introduction

Hello, my name is Bob Dawson. My background has always been in health and social care. I qualified in mental health and learning disability nursing during the 1980s, working up to the level of nursing officer within the Health Service. I then moved as a senior manager into social care within the voluntary/charitable sector in 1991. Since then, I have been involved in education and development, consultancy and training, which became my full-time job from 1999.

My experiences of being involved in and providing training in the area of safeguarding include being a member of the multi-agency steering groups for the counties that used to be Avon 1998–2000, being at the launch of *No Secrets*, being at the launch of *Making Safeguarding Personal*. Writing and delivering cross-agency training programmes for a variety of local authorities including South Gloucestershire, Bath and North East Somerset, North Somerset, Bristol City and Somerset. Developing and delivering bespoke training programmes for a multitude of specific organisations and groups including Milestones, Visions, Thornleigh Camphill Communities Ltd, Aspirations, and Headway, trustees, dentists, doctors, South Gloucestershire Football Association and housing associations.

I have also been a member of various safeguarding adult groups and training subgroups.

These training programmes covered areas including raising concerns (one/two-day course for all staff in health and social care and support services), management roles (one day course for social workers and seniors and managers and above in health and social care and support services) and identifying and preventing organisational abuse (one day course for managers and above in relevant health and social care agencies). All courses were aimed at developing a safeguarding profile within individual teams.

I have chosen the most frequently asked questions from these training programmes to form the book's index. This publication aims to replicate a variety of training sessions.

This is not an academic publication. It is aimed at anyone involved in health and social care, including family members and the general public. Some of the information is anecdotal, coming from over 40 years of experience working in the area and from the many people I have trained during this time.

Before you start looking for the answers to your questions, this is a generic book going across all local authorities. You need to be aware of your local multi-agency policy and your own agency's policy for specific responses, such as contact points, thresholds for reporting and responsibilities for reporting, which can be obtained via the local authority website (the local authority safeguarding board website normally contains the multi-agency policy and procedures), or by direct telephone contact. I also believe most staff practice at a high level of good practice and hope many reading this book will be saying, 'We already do that.' Excellent, but remember, no matter how good your practice is it can also be better. I hope you find something new here to stimulate you and your team to that better practice.

While this book is written using legislation applicable in England and Wales, the principles are universal.

To keep you up to date with further information I request you only read information from reputable resources who check the authenticity of information they put on their various websites. A list of these organisations in the UK are included in the appendix at the end of this book.

Most of my experience comes from interactions with staff from health and social care settings. However, I feel there is a value to this book for families and members of the general public, in that it gives an awareness of what regulations and standards are set in this important area, therefore giving a better understanding of how and why staff are using safeguarding procedures. Also, in establishing their role, and what they should do, if they have concerns.

Your questions answered

1. What is the difference between safeguarding procedures and good practice?

This is an interesting question, which always results in a lively debate. If we start with the realisation that safeguarding enquiries rarely occur where there is evidence of good practice, I would therefore state that good practice is one antidote to poor safeguarding in organisational abuse. I also recognise that good practice includes the reporting of concerns across all aspects of safeguarding, both within and out with an individual service.

Most teams and individuals already operate using good practice. I hope that for many of you this book reaffirms your good practice, and you are saying we already do that. I also hope you find one or two suggestions you are not already doing and add them to your practice to make it even safer, remember the aim is always to improve no matter how good your practice is. I am also aware that there are many teams and individuals whose practice is not as safe as it should be. If you are not doing something that is suggested in this book, don't see it as a criticism, see it as a challenge to improve your individual and/or your team's good practice.

You may find it useful to see safeguarding as an iceberg. One tenth lies above the surface, see this as the reactive side of safeguarding, what policies say we must do if we suspect abuse has happened. Nine tenths of the iceberg lie beneath the surface, rarely seen but vital in the life of the iceberg. See this part as proactive safeguarding, good practice that makes the likelihood of abuse less. I would therefore argue that adult safeguarding is the legal system laid down as part of the Care Act 2014 that explains how we should deal with all reports of adult abuse across the country, and good practice is the system by which we reduce the likelihood of adult abuse occurring.

2. What happened before *No Secrets* 1999?

I hope you will find it useful to start with a very brief history lesson to better understand why it took so long in this country to start showing more respect and balance towards certain marginalised groups. Specifically, here, people with learning difficulties, mental health and epilepsy. Thanks in part to the eugenics movement, we saw large groups of people deemed undesirable to society excluded into institutions during the 1800s and 1900s. These groups were devalued, disrespected, and not afforded rights available in 'normal' society. It is also worth pointing out that there were many other marginalised groups in society who were not institutionalised: these included older adults, people with physical disabilities and those with drug and alcohol dependencies to name a few.

While it is painful reading, there is a lot available to set the picture of life within the institution (for example, Getting it right together – Unit 3 – A history of learning disabilities, Helen Atherton, Lecturer in Learning Disabilities, University of Hull).

Several reports and changes in legislation sounded the end of the institutions. These included: 1959 Mental Health Act (ended compulsory certification enabling the discharge of many people with learning disabilities from long term institutions), 1971 white paper – Better Services for the Mentally Handicapped (advocated a 50% reduction in hospital places by 1991, and an increase in the provision of local-authority-based residential and day care) and in 1979 the Jay Report (re-emphasised the need for local-authority-led care and, importantly, a service philosophy based on the provision of normalisation).

Prior to 1999 there was no specific government guidance in relation to adult safeguarding. One consequence of this lack of guidance was that some individuals and organisations failed to share information that may have prevented or stopped abuse, and often resulted in action not being taken against abusers. This was partly because of a failure to understand the difference between confidentiality and secrets. Hence the need for *No Secrets*. When I started working in health care in the late 70s, most care was state based with NHS hospitals and large institutions for people with mental health issues, learning disability and epilepsy. Most social care provision was run by the local authority, a real difference from today where there is now a myriad of care providers, in addition to health and local authority services in the charitable, voluntary and private sectors. From the mid-1960s onwards the move from institutional care towards community care started to gather pace. By 1999 most of the large institutions for people with learning disability, mental health and epilepsy were closed, the land they occupied sold, and are now mainly housing developments for the general population. It is interesting to note that the amount and scale of provision, particularly for older people and those with dementia, was and is still increasing since 1999.

Within the state-driven system there was a very insular approach with each setting sorting out problems internally with no legal requirement to do otherwise, except for criminal legislation. This resulted in little sharing of information across boundaries and a culture of not sharing information internally. This was in part created by the hierarchical systems in place, lack of observation of practice by external people, especially in the institutions, poor staff to service user ratios, by little meaningful training about responsibilities to raise concerns and by general society's attitude towards raising concerns and reporting colleagues. There was, and to some extent there still is, a misunderstanding of what confidentiality means. This means that many professionals did not pass on relevant information either internally with colleagues, or externally, due to their belief that it was breaking the service user's right for confidentiality.

It is important to state that most staff working in the long-stay institutions were honourable people doing the best they could with difficult environments and poor staffing levels. Many were campaigning for a change in living environments, better staffing levels and an end to the segregation of individuals from society. Good staff with good practice always safeguarded individuals they had a responsibility for.

It took several significant reports into abuse happening in the sector to move societal and political thinking into ending the institutional management of these individuals. The most significant of these being the 'Report of the Committee of Enquiry into Ely Hospital' (Howe Report 1969).

3. What has changed since *No Secrets* 1999 was implemented?

It is important to stress that *No Secrets* was issued as a guidance document under Section 7 of the Social Work Act. This meant that local authorities would have their compliance assessed as part of their statutory inspection processes. However, there were no legal requirements; this was a guidance document.

I was at the launch of *No Secrets* at Warwick University in 1999, as part of the councils who used to be Avon multi-agency safeguarding group, and well remember the then health secretary John Denham introducing the document as a revenue neutral document!

On the front cover of *No Secrets* it stated, 'Guidance on developing and implementing multi-agency policies and procedures to protect vulnerable adults from abuse'.

It established six categories of abuse. These were physical, sexual, psychological, financial or material, neglect and acts of omission, and discriminatory abuse.

It established the local authority as the lead agency in adult safeguarding and required all other agencies operating in that local authority area to report all concerns about abuse to them.

It set out guidance on the following areas:

- Setting up an inter-agency framework.
- Developing inter-agency policy.
- Procedures for responding in individual cases.
- Getting the message across.

No Secrets also detailed the requirement to ensure training across the workforce to meet the need for the developing policies in this area.

During the period 1999–2014 we saw the setting up of multi-agency policies and procedures, internal policies in each individual organisation, the start of safeguarding adult boards, the development of a training matrix covering the variety of training needs across the health and social care workforce, the establishment of safeguarding teams within the local authority covering both individual abuse and later organisational abuse teams, the development of advocacy services for the person allegedly abused.

Each of the above areas developed as more agencies came on board. The difference between the early systems in 1999 and those in 2014 was dramatic, and has shown both the professionalism of those involved and the real value of multi-agency involvement. Vast improvements for service users were further enhanced by the launch of *Making Safeguarding Personal* guide in 2014. (See question 5.)

4. Who does safeguarding affect?

Safeguarding is everyone's responsibility. From all social and health care/support staff to members of the public to families, friends, other service users and strangers. It does not matter who you are, if you see or hear something that makes you concerned abuse may be a factor, you must not keep this to yourself. I want you to see every concern, no matter how small or seemingly insignificant, as a jigsaw piece; it may help build a picture based on other information available. Your jigsaw piece may be the one that completes the picture. Every local authority has a website where you can find relevant telephone numbers to report concerns. Every social and health care/support service in each local authority area has their own safeguarding policy and there is the multi-agency policy giving clear guidelines about reporting concerns. Do not forget, if you think you may have witnessed or been told about a potential crime, the police should also be notified as well.

5. What is the impact of *Making Safeguarding Personal* 2014?

I was at the launch of Making Safeguarding Personal 2014 at Orc House in London as part of a group from South Gloucestershire Social Services, South Gloucestershire having been one of the pilot sites for this report.

In essence, *Making Safeguarding Personal* is the guide that ensures the person who has allegedly been abused is at the centre of their own safeguarding. That they are involved, informed, their views sought, and actions taken, where possible, based on their wishes. It is:

- *A shift in culture and practice in response to what we now know about what makes safeguarding more effective from the perspective of the person being safeguarded.*
- *About having conversations with people about how we might respond in safeguarding situations in a way that enhances involvement, choice and control as well as improving quality of life, wellbeing and safety.*
- *About collecting information about the extent to which this shift has a positive impact on people's lives.*
- *A shift from a process supported by conversations to a series of conversations supported by a process. (Making safeguarding Personal Guide 2014.)*

Background.

'We have found, through peer challenges and other work that without a person-centred approach:

- Whilst they appreciate the work of individual staff, people tend to feel driven through a process in safeguarding. At best they are involved rather than in control, at worst they are lucky if they are kept informed about what professionals are doing.
- Some people want access to some form of justice or resolution, such as through criminal or civil law, or restorative justice, or through knowing that some form of disciplinary or other action has been taken. They may feel disappointed or let down if this does not happen.
- Some people have no wish for any formal proceedings to be pursued and may be distressed when this happens without their knowledge or agreement.
- What we have monitored as outputs have tended to centre on such things as decisions about whether abuse was substantiated or not and what was done as a result: often additional services or monitoring.
- Whilst most people do want to be safer, other things may be as, or more, important: maintaining relationships is an obvious one. We know from a national prevalence study that; Where people have been subject to financial abuse ... respondents commonly viewed the financial loss to be less significant than the emotional and psychological impacts. For example, respondents could suffer low self-esteem and blame themselves for having "let" themselves be taken advantage of.' (Making Safeguarding Personal Guide, 2014)

I thought it useful to replicate this part of the guide here as it sets the scene as to why it was and is necessary. Up to then, safeguarding was the property of the professionals, not the abused. How often did the individual allegedly abused attend or in any way participate in their own safeguarding meetings, what say did they have in the outcome of their own safeguarding? Since 2014 it is becoming increasingly rare for the abused person not to be involved or represented in their strategy meeting and be involved in their updates throughout the process. Especially where there are capacity issues, the use of advocacy services for the individual have dramatically increased as this is now a requirement under the Care Act guidance.

Making Safeguarding Personal does not ease the responsibility to report, even if the person wants you to take no further action (see question 20). It does not interfere with the safeguarding process or the multi-agency involvement including police involvement. It ensures that the action taken in the process considers the individuals views seriously, and where possible their views are listened to and acted on.

'What good is it making someone safer if it merely makes them miserable?' (Local Authority X v MM &Anor (No 1) (2007) Lord Justice Mumby, Supreme Court.)

6. What has changed since the Care Act 2014 was implemented?

Appendix 2 at the end of the book gives the website details for the Care Act 2014. Here I will give a brief account of the main changes that took place when the act became law in April 2015 and adult safeguarding became a legal requirement.

The Care Act 2014 was based on developing good practice coming from the work performed in this area since *No Secrets* was introduced. *No Secrets* was replaced by the act along with most previous law regarding carers and people being cared for.

Three new categories of abuse were added to those in *No Secrets*. These are modern slavery, self-neglect and domestic violence or abuse. The category of institutional abuse was changed to organisational abuse. Interestingly, six years on many staff are still unaware of some of these changes. Why?

The local authority must lead a multi-agency local adult safeguarding system (lead agency), and was given the legal duty to make enquiries or ensure others do so where a concern is raised or suspected. They must also carry out safeguarding adult reviews where they are deemed appropriate, and arrange for an independent advocate, if required.

There are three criteria laid down and it is the responsibility of the local authority to decide whether or not referrals have met these criteria:

1. The person has needs for care and support (whether the authority is meeting any of those needs). Unfortunately, the Care Act does not specify what these are, therefore local interpretation may vary.
2. The person is experiencing, or is at risk of, abuse or neglect, and
3. As a result of those needs the person is unable to protect themselves against the abuse or neglect or the risk of it.

Safeguarding adults boards were put on a legal status. (See question 14.)

The local authority must cooperate with each of its relevant partners to protect adults experiencing or at risk of abuse.

The term vulnerable adult was replaced by adult/person at risk. Personally, I think this is a great change as it means we now must risk-assess and quantify the risk to the individual instead of just labelling them as vulnerable, which often left the staff unclear as to why and what that meant for both the individual and for themselves as staff. This also prevented some service users being allowed to take acceptable risks because of their perceived yet unquantified vulnerability.

The word investigation was dropped and replaced by enquiries.

The term alert has been replaced by raising a concern.

The Social Care Institute for Excellence (SCIE) has developed valuable information in this area, on their website (Appendix 2) for all stakeholders in safeguarding. This information includes guidance in a wide range of areas from sharing information to gaining access, from practice questions to prevention and wellbeing and much more. If you are not already registered with SCIE then I would strongly recommend you do so. Over many years they have been supplying excellent information to aid development of good practice in a wide range of areas.

7. What are the six key principles of the Care Act 2014?

Empowerment – Are people supported and encouraged to make their own decisions? How has this been done? For example, are you making services more personal, giving people choice and control over decisions, and are you asking people what they want the outcome to be?

What does this mean to the adult? – You are asked what you want to happen and services plan safeguarding around this.

Protection – Your organisations must ensure that all staff know what to do when abuse has happened, all involved know what to do if there are concerns, how to stop the abuse and how to offer help and support for people at risk.

What does this mean for the adult? – You get help and support to tell people about abuse and can get involved in the safeguarding as much or as little as you want.

Prevention – Your organisation does work together with relevant people to stop abuse before it happens, by raising awareness about abuse and neglect, staff training and making sure clear, simple and accessible information is available about abuse and where people can get help.

What does this mean for the adult? – You get clear and simple information about what abuse is and who to ask for help.

Proportionality – When dealing with abuse situations, services must ensure that they always think about risk. Any response should be appropriate to the risk presented. Services must respect the person, think about what is best for them and only get involved as much as needed.

What does this mean for the adult? – Services think about what is best for you, where possible agree with you and only get involved when they need to.

Partnership – Organisations should work in partnership with each other and local communities. Local people also have a part to play in preventing, detecting and reporting abuse.

What does this mean for the adult? – Staff look after your personal information and only share it when this helps to keep you safe.

Accountability – Safeguarding is everybody's business. Everyone must accept that we are all accountable as individuals, services and as organisations. Roles and responsibilities are clear so that people can see and check how safeguarding is done.

What does this mean for the adult? – You know what all the different people should do to keep you safe.

What are you doing with the six core principles? How do they sit within your service? Have you checked your service against them and prepared an action plan of possible improvements based on them? This may be something to share with inspectors to show your service is proactive in its development. The above suggestions are not exhaustive and hopefully you can be creative to ensure you match the principles to your service.

8. What are the different categories of abuse?

Physical abuse.
Sexual abuse.
Emotional or psychological abuse.
Organisational abuse (previously institutional abuse, renamed in the Care Act 2014)

Neglect or acts of omission.
Self-neglect (added by the Care Act 2014).
Financial or material abuse.
Domestic violence or abuse (added by the Care Act 2014).
Modern slavery (added by the Care Act 2014).
Discriminatory abuse.

This is according to the Care Act, not an exhaustive list. Across the country there are different words used. My rule of thumb has always been that if you feel someone is being badly treated, that should be enough to report further.

Do you know what fits into each category? Has your team discussed the categories in relation to your service and your responsibilities? In question 13 step 2, I have asked your manager to go through the categories of abuse to establish a team value base. Please be supportive of this and the other steps. If your team has identified what is unacceptable practice and given each other permission to raise concerns in these areas, then abuse is already less likely. Why would a colleague use unacceptable practice when they had already given you permission to take it further?

Let's partially break down two areas, financial or material abuse and physical abuse, to see what it may start to look like.

Financial or material abuse. Imagine you were working in a domiciliary care/support team, your list may look something like:

- Stealing money or possessions.
- Accepting gifts/presents beyond what your organisations policy allows.
- Using your loyalty card when purchasing items for your service user.
- When shopping keeping the get one free when purchasing items for your service user.
- Putting pressure on individuals to purchase items which you benefit from and they don't, e.g., streaming services.

In some services this may be a long list, in others where you have no control over finance or property it may be very short.

Physical abuse. Imagine you are working in a 50-bedded nursing home, your list may look something like:

- Hitting.
- Spitting.
- Grabbing and bruising.
- Poor manual handling.
- Kicking.
- Not following agreed procedures for mobility equipment.

Again, in some services this may be a long list, but where you are supporting people who do not have physical disabilities it may be a short list.

9. Who can abuse?

Anyone can abuse, very few do. In terms of safeguarding there are different groups of abusers. For example, staff abusing service user, family members abusing their at-risk family member. Family and friends acting as unpaid carers could be both perpetrators and victims, especially where either has cognitive impairment and does not fully understand the consequences of their actions. Significant others in the at-risk person's network. Service users at risk, or not, abusing at-risk service users. Strangers not known to the at-risk person. In organisational abuse, staff (often including policies and procedures) and multiple at-risk service users.

For the purpose of this book, I want to delve further into problems occurring where staff are implicated as the abuser. Where the abuse is by one person against the other and does not involve staff, we find this easier to deal with. I am not diluting the impact on the abused and others close to them, but I am stating that within the team we remain more professional, and the impact is less traumatic on other staff members. Why? I can only assume this is because none of our team are implicated, and therefore we are able to work through the situation with our energies concentrated on supporting the allegedly abused. When we choose to work with people at risk it is to help and support them, and we find it hard to believe, or understand, how others do not have the same beliefs.

However, where it is alleged that one staff member has abused a service user in our service, especially when the reporting has been done by a work colleague, then the impact on the staff team can be profound. Why? Again, I can only assume the impact of 'one of our own' being involved is difficult to understand. Some staff may believe they could not possibly have done such a thing, while others are in shock that such an event could have happened within their team.

I am asking each manager to sit down with their team and have a conversation about relevant policies, and discuss how they would cope if such an event ever happened within their services. What the process would be, what would be the role of individual members of the team? What communications would be allowed during this process? We must move beyond shock to planned contingency. I have worked with teams who could not work together after a traumatic safeguarding enquiry because of the trauma caused to the team. A lot of this trauma was caused be staff not knowing what would happen during this period and feeling let down by the process.

One of the major problems of safeguarding accusations is that it happens so infrequently within each team. While this is excellent, it does mean teams are often not prepared: they have no fall-back strategy to deal with the situation. In many cases they start developing their strategies after the abuse has been reported. I am not talking about the safeguarding system; it is laid down in each local authority area and will run its course once the concern has activated the need for the implementation of safeguarding procedures. I am talking about the internal systems within a team regarding what will happen next and communication protocols, how safeguarding may affect ongoing day-to-day working, relationships within the staff team during this period and so on. These should already have been discussed prior to a major safeguarding enquiry so the staff team know, clearly, what is expected of them during the ongoing enquiry.

Safeguarding should not be a taboo subject within the staff team. It should be maturely planned for in the hope that this planning will never be needed. We already do similar planning around events like fire. We have complex systems including drills so that all staff involved know what to do in the unlikely event of a fire breaking out in our workplaces. However, most of us will never experience a severe fire in our workplace. Therefore, we must recognise that risk assessment and management should not be merely a reactive tool, i.e. putting things in place after things have gone wrong, but a more proactive tool to be used to minimise the risk of harm. To this end in safeguarding, we need to be better prepared, not just organisationally, but on a team-to-team basis.

The next three questions are ones I always ask in basic raising-concerns training. They are aimed at encouraging participants to expose and discuss the main issues in adult safeguarding as they affect them in their day-to-day work. The group is split into three and given flipchart paper and pens. Each group is given a different question and given 20 minutes to come up with answers to the questions. While this basic training is mandatory for all staff, most staff attending any session will be comprised of junior staff.

10. What might you witness, hear, discover that you need to take further?

This is the question for the first group. I ask them not to state the obvious, i.e. abuse which they believe breaches any of the categories of abuse (level 3 report, see question 13, step 3). I get them to agree that such breaches are automatic reports to social services using set safeguarding procedures within their workplace and multi-agency policies and procedures.

Instead, I ask them to think about anything that has in the past or might in the future make them feel uncomfortable in their work setting (levels 1 and 2, see question 13, step 3). The most common areas raised include: someone, whether staff or family, speaking on behalf of the service user when they are quite capable of speaking for themselves, patronising behaviour, attitude of care givers including family, controlling behaviour, smells and odours.

What I am aiming to do with this question is to open those areas that cause us to feel uncomfortable often long before we suspect abuse, and explore what if anything should be done about them. Many participants agree they may do nothing more than keep an eye on the situation. Equally, many agree that they would make a record of all concerns and talk them through with a colleague/supervisor/manager. As a basic rule of thumb, I encourage all participants that no member of staff should take a concern home by themselves without recording and sharing. It is by early identification of potential problems and sharing of concerns that we are more likely to reduce the risk of abuse; this should be seen as good practice. Obviously, sharing of information and who you should speak to should be in line with your policy on sharing information.

It is clear to me that this remains a problem area in many teams. Has your team discussed, and agreed, what you should share, when should you share it and to whom?

Let me give you examples frequently raised at this point to illustrate this area as one of potential weakness in many teams:

Professional staff visiting service users in their own homes, stating that they feel uncomfortable when family members speak on behalf of the service user, not giving them the opportunity to speak for themselves or speaking over them. Many staff talk about feeling uncomfortable with behaviours of other staff, e.g. being too abrupt, moody, too direct in their dealings with the service users, but then say they have always been like that – that is just who they are! Cutting corners to get the task done more quickly. Overly regimented routines. Others talk about having a feeling or an intuition that something is wrong, but have little to support their concern. Some raise what they see as unhealthy attitudes from either family members or other staff, including comments like being too defensive at suggestions, not listening or following advice.

With all the above examples and many more I always give the same answer. Doing nothing is unacceptable. If appropriate, have you raised your concern with the individual involved? Have you raised it in supervision? Have you had a chat with a senior or even colleague to talk through your concerns? Remember, the most important thing is not to have your concern only in your head; if you are correct and something is wrong, how bad will you feel if you did nothing?

We also cover what all staff should do if they suspect abuse that breaches any of the categories of abuse (level 3). Report. Record. Review.

Report as per your policy, usually to a senior or line manager.

Record dated and signed. Giving relevant details of suspected abuse.

Review. This initial review covers what has happened to the concern you have raised. Has it been passed on to the local authority safeguarding team or not? If not, have you been given reasons that satisfy you? If not, what does your policy say you should do in terms of escalating the policy or whistleblowing (see question 22)?

As a manager, have you discussed with and given permission to your staff to escalate the policy, and are you confident that they would do so?

11. What systems in place where you work are aimed at reducing the risk of abuse occurring?

The most common answers are policies and procedures including supervision, training, care/support plans, risk assessments, finance, safeguarding, communication systems such as running records and handovers, record keeping and recruitment.

All these systems are mandatory in health and social care and support services, however, it is clear that having the systems is not enough; ongoing evaluation of their effectiveness and continued development is essential to ensure good practice is ongoing and improving.

Let me pull apart some of these systems to explain what I mean.

Supervision – We are aware that when good supervision is in place it is easier for staff to pass on concerns at an earlier stage. We discuss what comprises good supervision and come up with a list including trust, relationship with supervisor being constructive, space and time allocated, sharing of agendas and discussing things relevant to both parties. Mutual growth and development of both supervisor and supervisee. I then challenge each participant to look at their own supervision and see if there is anything, they could do to improve it when they return to work.

Given the number of staff I have seen over many years there are a few points I would be negligent not to mention here. While it is obvious that many staff enjoy good supervision, many do not. Supervision should not be done just because it is a requirement (even though it is!).

For too many staff, supervision is merely a tick box exercise or an opportunity for a manager to 'instruct'. There is a need to look closely and give clearer guidelines where the supervisor and supervisee can only meet irregularly, such as in domiciliary care.

Where there is a large staff team comprising several different grades of staff more consideration needs to be given as to who the supervisor should be to ensure the person being supervised is not left in a power imbalance situation. I would be radical enough to suggest that good supervision is one of the natural antidotes to abuse. Done well it encourages involvement, it greatly enhances communication, and it encourages staff to share concerns often before there is a major problem. Another antidote, where it works well, is group supervision – sharing ideas with peers can help people check out their thinking and values.

I always found in my own clinical practice that good supervision saved time. From the feedback I receive during these sessions there is still a lot of work to be done in many areas to improve supervision. I always enjoy the part of the session where staff who are receiving good supervision try to persuade those who are not about the benefits of good supervision, not only for the individuals concerned but also for the team and the service. It is wonderful to watch a group training themselves and not just being led by the trainer. If managed well it is one of the real benefits of multi-agency training.

Training – One of my major concerns, and one shared by safeguarding adults boards, is the quality of training available in this area. After speaking to many participants their previous training ranges from a half-hour video to an open learning e-package with no follow up. This training remains uncertified apart from the attendance certificate.

I am aware when carrying out training for different local authorities of the number of agencies who do not send staff for multi-agency training. While this training is mandatory, the guidance from the Care Quality Commission is that managers are required to ensure that staff are adequately trained in this area. But it is also that manager's responsibility to check on the content and quality of that training and how it is followed up in the workplace.

I have attended conferences over the years where trainers

discuss the content and other aspects of safeguarding training and am aware of many excellent training providers in this area. As a trainer training local authority staff, I am frequently 'observed' by members of the management team, safeguarding board and training managers to ensure the training is meeting acceptable standards. We are also subject to evaluation forms at the end of each session completed by each participant, which are collated by the training team, and feedback given to us as trainers.

However, I do have real concerns about the number of staff who may not be adequately trained and organisations who do not see the necessity for high standards of training in this area. It is surely time for minimum standards to be set in this area on a national basis.

As a manager, are you training staff just to meet statutory requirements, ticking the box, or is training a way of developing and improving practice? At least twice a month, often more, participants turn up for the mandatory raising adult safeguarding concerns training course ask to see the registration list, as they were only told the where and when of the training but not the course. Does your system have a pre-training requirement and a post training evaluation, looking at changes of practice based on the training? Is the trainer evaluated as providing training suitable to your service? How is this done? What systems are you using as a manager to ensure training is positively affecting practice? Do you re-evaluate the impact of the training say three months after the training to plot improvements in good practice?

Risk assessments. The change brought in by the Care Act 2014 to change the term 'vulnerable adult' to 'person at risk' impacts here. Personally, I had great problems with the word vulnerable as it was often used as an umbrella term to describe individuals within certain groups, for example learning disability, elderly, and people with capacity issues. But in speaking to staff, they could rarely define what vulnerable meant in relation to the individual so labelled. They would come up with general terms such as frail, weak, and unable to make decisions. With the new title 'person at risk' there is now a need to define the risk and quantify how it should be managed. This should make it much easier for staff to be more informed about their responsibilities in these areas and allow for increased prevention in this area. Of course, risk assessments should be completed with the person at risk's involvement, and take into account their viewpoint where possible.

Have your paperwork systems been updated to show this change? How do you monitor and record ongoing risk?

As managers you should identify all the policies and procedures within your service that aim to minimise the risk of abuse and check there are monitoring systems and that they are known to all staff and working.

12. Why may some staff and others not report suspected abuse?

The group is asked not to speak from their own value base but to reflect on reasons those who do not report may give. As you will know if you have read any adult case review (carried out as part of the review procedure after the abuse has been dealt with), there will be a paragraph stating that had staff shared their concerns earlier then in some cases the abuse may have been prevented, and in others it may have been stopped much earlier. These are the most common responses groups give:

- Lack of training.
- Too busy.
- Not sure if it is abuse or not.
- Above my pay grade, that's the responsibility of the qualified staff.
- Lack of communication in our team.
- Frightened of my manager.
- Don't want myself/my friend/relative to get into trouble.

- Lack of continuity of care.
- Nobody will do anything.
- Don't care.
- Those that work closest with the person should do it. I only see them once a week.
- I work in domiciliary care and do not speak to my manager/supervisor regularly.
- Don't want to put my head above the parapet.
- Don't want to create an atmosphere in the team.
- My system is hierarchical, and I would be frightened to report someone much more senior than me.
- Told not to.
- Fear of victimisation/losing my job/poor reference.

While I would like to believe that the majority of those who attend training would report, it is scary how easily they come up with these answers. There is certainly anecdotal evidence based on the thousands of staff I have trained that problems with reporting are more likely to occur in the following situations. Where there is a hierarchical system. Where there are basic communication issues, such as in some domiciliary services there is little face-to-face contact between staff, this is becoming an increasing problem in some supported living services. It is important to recognise that there is some excellent practice in some of these areas where managers have risk-assessed this issue and put measures in place to limit the effects of the problems created by the service.

This question highlights problems with reporting and shows up some current issues that should not be ignored. For example, comments like 'lack of training'; training in this area is mandatory but does your current training cover issues specific to your service? 'Lack of communication' highlights poor management. 'Don't care' stimulates healthy discussion, but most groups agree that there are a small group of staff in the health and social care sector who have no affinity with the client group they are working with, and they are only in the job for financial reasons. In some cases, it is felt this can lead to a higher level of detachment and a feeling of less responsibility to doing the right thing. Another area to discuss within 'don't care' is burn out, has this been considered?

Other comments coming from staff working in hierarchical systems such as large nursing homes, NHS workers, and some domiciliary and supported living workers, need to be taken seriously and discussed in team settings where clear responsibilities and protocols can be developed. Most importantly, clear permission and protection is agreed for the concerned member of staff to raise concerns without prejudice to themselves. This would be assisted quickly by all staff being aware of escalation/ whistleblowing policies and being made to feel safe in using them. (See question 22.)

For managers, see the six steps to enhance good practice, step five deals specifically with this issue (question 13).

13. Six steps exercise for managers and staff teams to enhance good practice.

After 21 years of developing training programmes and training staff in health and social care staff in adult safeguarding, I have developed a six-step process to ensure the building blocks of good practice for individual teams are solid. If managers put all six steps in place, their systems will be more robust and safer. Remember, if your practice is already good, and many are, it can and should be better.

It is my sincere hope that safeguarding managers, Care Quality Commission inspectors, commissioners of services, contract managers, internal organisation auditors/inspection teams, trustees and any other monitors of service delivery find a way to incorporate this six-step process into their existing tools to check the effectiveness of the safeguarding/promotion of good practice in individual services.

Most teams in health and social care settings are already operating to a high level of good practice within adult safeguarding. Some of the common factors in these teams are: good and visible management, good communication systems including supervision, good training which encourages staff, of all grades, to share concerns and have a learning and development culture which embraces the development of individual staff.

Step 1. Safeguarding Folder

Each team should have a safeguarding folder, or equivalent, which aims to ease the paperwork process when a safeguarding referral is required. One of the biggest problems with the process is that in some teams a referral is infrequent, and staff are not fluent in its use. With proper planning we should have safeguarding on the same focus as fire. Something we rarely, if ever, have to deal with, but all know how to do so professionally. This folder should contain: – the local authority policy and procedures, example copies of the paperwork for the local authority/CQC, relevant legislation that staff may need to consider.

Many staff have said to me that they were required to fill in forms for the local authority that they had never seen or used before, for example the raising concerns form. Each team should identify who may be required to complete such information, and on-the-job training should be given during, say, supervision. A blank copy of the local authority strategy meeting notes and so on. Remember, you will be judged by what you should have done, not necessarily just on what you have done. The reporting of abuse is often a time where emotions are raised; we need to plan and prepare to ensure we act professionally.

I have described the reactive side of adult safeguarding, from a technical point of view, as boring. This is not to take away anything from the situation, however, our responsibility is to report, record and review. Pass the information on to the local authority and other relevant agencies on pre-set paperwork and then work collectively to minimise or remove the risk of future abuse. There is no place at this time for innovation or lone working but a need to follow the laid down process and make sure the person is safe. Therefore, there is no reason why with effective planning and preparation the process should be reasonably clear and easily followed by all staff.

Step 2. Team Value Base

To assume all staff will have the same value base and will report concerns at the same time is naïve. Each member of staff is a unique individual with their own belief system, pressures and perceptions. This exercise forms a team value base and eliminates the ability of individual staff to operate outside of the team value base without consequences.

At a handover staff meeting, go through the categories of abuse, (question 8), concentrating on those most relevant to your service. Invite your staff to state unacceptable practice in each area (level 3 see step 3 below). Compile a list of all areas agreed as unacceptable. Remember, you are looking for areas which you would expect staff to report to a senior because they believe this to be abuse. When you finish the list ask staff if they saw any of these happening, or if they were told about them, what would they do? Encourage them to say Report (to a senior, or to the local authority safeguarding team), Record and Review. Compile the list showing how staff agreed they should react, and you now have a completed team value base. This exercise takes away the ability of staff to say they did not know they should report those areas included in the team value base. The exercise should be recorded and all staff in the team asked to sign it.

For this exercise to work well you need to prepare for this and be able to prompt staff to areas they may not have thought of. If it is difficult to get the whole team together then do it in two or perhaps three stages, each new group adding to what the last group agreed. Remember this list is for those areas where it is considered abuse might have taken place and should be reported further.

Step 3. Three Levels of Reporting

How do you promote, as a manager, staff to share concerns about poor practice and not just wait until it becomes so bad that they eventually report because they feel it is now abuse based on what was agreed in the team value base?

By introducing the three levels of reporting into your team you will start the process where staff feel more comfortable in raising concerns early, at the point they first have them. This is best introduced to staff via supervision and then through team discussions. Level 3 is straight forward as you will already have identified relevant areas in your team's value base. However, in improving good practice and further reducing the risk of abuse level 1 and 2 are key.

Level 1. When something happens to challenge a staff members value base by, for example, a service users relative or colleague, such as, cutting corners, speaking over someone, poor manual handling, speaking abruptly or rudely, not promoting independence, not offering choice properly, staff should challenge the person where possible and safe. Would your staff feel comfortable raising a concern with a colleague within your team or a service users family member? If not, why would this be a problem? Have you discussed this with staff during supervision?

If it is not possible to raise their concern with the individual concerned, they should move directly to level 2 and raise it with a more senior member of staff. What staff say at level 1 where they are confronting a service user's relative or a colleague will depend on where they are on the assertiveness scale. If they are very passive and any conflict puts a knot in their stomach, they may only say, 'Are you having a bad day?' If they are in the middle of the assertiveness scale, they may say, 'Have you tried doing it like this' or, 'If I was doing this I would do it this way', and if they were at the top of the assertiveness scale they may say, 'That made me feel uncomfortable, if that happens again, I will need to take it further.' Staff during supervision should be encouraged to discuss where they are on the assertiveness scale and how they may react to witnessing poor practice.

Level 2. If the staff need to speak to someone who is displaying poor practice more than once and nothing changes, then staff should automatically share their concerns with someone more senior. We should not be waiting for behaviour to deteriorate to levels where abuse is more likely before dealing with it. As a manager you will need to have developed systems to deal with level 2 concerns that make staff feel that they have done the right thing by coming to see you. Your ability to deal with practice issues like these will require sensitivity and skill, otherwise staff may be reluctant to raise further concerns. With every group I have trained I give them two options and ask them to choose one of them. Please feel free to use these options with your staff team. Option one: when one of our colleagues is behaving inappropriately, we should keep a diary of all the things they are not doing well, and when we have enough evidence we should present this to our manager for you to deal with. Or option two: when we see a colleague doing something inappropriate, where possible we should point it out to them. If they continue as before we should then raise it with more senior staff at supervision, or discretely after handover. Every participant goes for option 2. But is this what is happening in your team? How do you monitor this? Also, every participant at training agrees that they would rather a colleague come directly if they were doing something that is causing concern, rather than going to their manager/supervisor.

Level 3. Is a line drawn in the sand, where behaviour is believed to be unacceptable as identified in the team value base, and therefore potentially abusive? Here all staff should report directly to a senior or the local authority safeguarding team. See your local and internal safeguarding policy to ensure you know your role in reporting suspected abuse. As a manager you need to be comfortable that each individual member of staff knows what is expected of them in this instance.

If you introduce the three levels of reporting successfully into your team you will be more likely to be on top of poor practice before it reaches level 3

Almost every Safeguarding Adults Review (SAR) contains comments like, 'Had staff shared their concerns at the point they first became concerned in some cases the abuse may not have happened, and in other cases it may have been stopped at a much earlier stage.' We must ensure that the trigger for staff raising concerns is not just some evidence of abuse happening but at the much earlier stage of poor practice.

Step 4. Manage Staff Expectations When Raising Concerns

Managers should ask their staff what they expect from them if they were to raise a safeguarding concern. There are three urban myths you may expose, detailed below, and give you the opportunity to discuss what is likely to happen if they raise a concern to you.

For many years I have been asking staff what they expect for more senior staff if they raise a safeguarding concern. Obvious answers include to be listened to, for managers to take their concerns further, to be believed, supported, kept informed, for the situation to be resolved and so on. Three of the most common answers however are unachievable in certain situations.

1. **Confidentiality.** Clearly this depends on the individuals understanding of this word. The fact that staff must record their concern and you must take this concern forward internally and externally already breaches many individuals understanding of the word confidentiality. Your legal guidance comes from the Public Interest Disclosure Act 1999 which clearly places two requirements

on you. Firstly, you will set up a need-to-know basis, immediately, and no-one else should be informed. Secondly, keeping the name of the person raising the concern away from the alleged perpetrator until the initial disciplinary or safeguarding enquiries are sufficient to be moving towards disciplinary or criminal action. At this point the alleged perpetrator has access to written reports so they can defend themselves.

It is important to note that no matter how strictly you adhere to these rules, it is not unusual for the alleged abuser to be aware of who was there when the alleged abuse happened or are aware of the worker's concerns and therefore works out quickly who has raised the concern.

There are still too many staff who believe confidentiality means no one will know they raised the concern.

2. **Support.** All staff expect the person who they raise concerns with will support them throughout the process. Where this is a staff-on-staff concern you may have an involvement in any potential disciplinary information gathering this will raise an obvious conflict of interest. In this situation you will not be able to support the person who raised the concern; however, it will remain your role to ensure they have access to support, but not from you. I have yet to meet a member of junior staff who knows this. There should be some discussion within the staff team as to who may offer this support. These discussions may involve others, such as area managers or human resources. All staff should be aware who may support them if you are unable to. Planning is so important as staff often feel let down by the system because of their own unrealistic perceptions about support which cannot happen.

3. **To be kept informed.** While this is logical and, in many cases correct, in one situation this is a real problem.

Where a member of staff reports a colleague in the same team and that individual is suspended, and after disciplinary investigation is believed to be safe to come back to work, little information can be shared. In fact, in most cases the most that can be shared is as follows. 'Thanks for sharing your concerns with me, I will be sharing this concern with the local authority safeguarding team and working with them, its ongoing.' And then eventually, 'This matter has now been dealt with using internal policies and procedures, if you think it's happening again come back and see me.' Most staff when I ask them if they want to know more say yes (about 99%). You need to introduce them to a new playing field, i.e., I raised a concern, it is no longer happening, it has been dealt with, or I raised a concern it, is still happening, I will raise it again. Obviously in many other situations you can give more information.

Teams need to discuss what information sharing might look like in a safeguarding situation. Including possible constraints on sharing information. This should be done as part of the planning process and not left until a safeguarding situation happens.

I worry that without this exercise being done some staff will continue to feel the system lets them down when they need it to support them because of their unrealistic expectations. This may in turn leave them less likely to use the system in the future.

Step 5. Problems With Staff Sharing Concerns

At a staff meeting ask staff for reasons they may find it difficult to raise concerns to you/other seniors with concerns they may have, either minor (level 2), or more serious (level 3).

Having personally asked this question over several years, typical answers are:

Don't want to get my friend into trouble. Don't want to create an atmosphere in the team. Not sure it has reached a stage where I need to report it. Not sure it's my responsibility. That's the qualified staff's job. Unsure of the policy and my responsibilities. Don't care, I'm only in the job to pay my bills.

Again, this exercise is aimed at making your team/service safer. For too long some managers have been sending their staff for safeguarding training without converting their learning to the workplace. Imagine the power of discussing the above reasons for not raising concerns within your team. Again, you need to prepare for this to prompt staff into areas they are not raising. If there are several senior staff that your team may be reporting to, you also need to ensure that there is consistency of approach among the senior staff. For example, if you work in a large nursing home, are you comfortable that a kitchen porter would be comfortable reporting a senior member of staff for poor practice at level 2? What systems have you in place that make you comfortable they would, and how are they monitored?

We need to put safeguarding on the agenda more frequently both from a reactive and a proactive point of view. There should be no secrets/surprises about the system that trip staff up because they were unaware or not prepared for them.

Step 6. Constructive Criticism

Please embed steps 1–5 before tackling this one. This step is unlikely to be effective unless the other steps are in place and working well. Steps 1–5 could easily be put in place over a 3–4 month period and are best done in the order they are laid out.

Constructive criticism is where each member of the team feels empowered to raise concerns with any colleague over a practice issue. Give your staff two options. If they were doing something which caused a colleague to feel concerned would they rather: A) that the staff member came to you and raised the concern for you to deal with (level 1), or B) would they hope they would approach them for a discussion about the practice causing concern (level 1). Every group I have given these options to has chosen option B.

I can assure you that this will not usually happen by some sort of natural process, but because staff within each team give each other permission to use constructive criticism in practice issues.

This is by far the hardest of the six steps and will require not just to be introduced at a staff meeting. There will need to be a careful discussion agreeing what is meant by practice issues and a careful monitoring and adjustments made as appropriate. For some teams, the normal reaction of an individual member of staff being criticised is to go on the offensive. Therefore, this is the last exercise and will only work well when the other five steps are in place and working well.

In conclusion it is time for safeguarding to be embedded into the heart of each team, for staff on a team-by-team basis to discuss safeguarding issues maturely and plan for eventualities that may well never happen, but if they do, they are prepared for them. We must stop ticking the box and saying all are staff are trained; managers need to demonstrate that safeguarding, and good practice, are a core responsibility within their team. The six steps will help to stimulate the process of team interaction, discussion, and further development in this core area.

14. What is the role of the safeguarding adult board?

Safeguarding adult boards were put on a legislative footing by the Care Act 2014.

Membership is set by the act as: the local authority, clinical commissioning group, chief police officer for the local authority and others as may be necessary for its function. This may include groups such as providers of services, contracts, training, advocacy services, probation, public health, NHS, and pharmacists.

They must develop and publish a strategic plan, publish an annual report and commission safeguarding adult reviews for any cases which meet the criteria for these.

Most groups meet 4–6 times a year.

The overarching purpose of the SAB is to help and safeguard adults with care and support needs. Typically, it does this by:

- Assuring itself that local safeguarding adult arrangements are in place as defined by the Care Act 2014 and statutory guidance.
- Assuring itself that safeguarding practice is person-centred and outcome focused.
- Working collaboratively to prevent abuse and neglect where possible.
- Ensuring agencies and individuals give timely and proportionate responses when abuse or neglect have occurred.
- Assuring itself that safeguarding practice is continuously improving and enhancing the quality of life of adults in this area.

After asking many staff who their representative on the SAB is, I am constantly surprised that less than 5% of those asked can answer correctly. You should recognise that the SAB is a strategic group of senior staff from many organisations across the local authority area overseeing this function.

Why may you need to contact your representative on the board? While there are many more reasons, two are worth commenting on here. Firstly, if you have been through safeguarding procedures situation and the system has worked well, sharing this with your representative may help speed learning from good practice to other services. Secondly, if you have been through safeguarding procedures and the system did not work properly, then sharing this with your representative may identify changes that improve the system for future cases.

Do you know who your representative on the SAB is? If not, go onto your local authority's website. Go onto their safeguarding section. Enter safeguarding adults board in the search box and you should find out who is on the board there.

15. What is the role of the local authority safeguarding team?

It is important for you to be familiar with the requirements laid down as part of your local multi-agency safeguarding policy and your own organisation's safeguarding policy.

The local authority safeguarding team is the initial point of contact, receiving all safeguarding referrals to the local authority. It is their responsibility to manage the criteria, laid down by the Care Act, all referrals are accepted, and then the decision is taken whether to progress to an enquiry. There is a legal requirement on all health and social care and support agencies to pass concerns on to the local authority where it is believed abuse may have occurred. However, you should never see your responsibility as being completed by just passing on your concern. Instead, you should see the passing on of the concern as starting a collaborative approach to resolve the issue(s) raised.

The local authority was given the legal duty to make enquiries or ensure others do so where a concern is raised. This means that in some cases the local authority will carry out the section 42 enquiry (see question 25), and in other cases they will ask the referring agency to carry out this enquiry and feed back to them. In all cases the local authority retains a responsibility until the risk is assessed and managed effectively or resolved.

Since 1999 when it became a requirement for all safeguarding cases to be reported to the local authority, a great level of expertise, professionalism and multi-agency collaboration has been developed within the teams receiving safeguarding referrals. We should see them as the experts in this field; remember their primary aim is to work with you to see the issue is resolved or professionally managed so that they no longer need to be involved.

16. Should I raise a concern, relative/member of the public?

Yes. Anyone who witnesses or hears something they are concerned may be abuse has a responsibility to take that concern further. Remember, safeguarding is everyone's responsibility. For social and health care/support staff this is a legal responsibility. For others this is a moral, ethical, civil duty. I would describe building a safeguarding case as like completing a jigsaw. Each piece or information represents another piece of the jigsaw. As the information builds, the picture becomes clearer. If everyone is not sharing their piece of the jigsaw, abuse may continue unchecked for much longer or go unnoticed.

I am not suggesting every concern should be reported to the local authority teams. For example, if you have a concern as a relative it may in the first instance be appropriate to talk about your concern with their care providers, who may be able to give you information that alleviates your concern, or act, if it is a poor practice issue, to your satisfaction.

If you are working, for example, in a dental, optician, audiology, mobility clinic and are concerned by the staff attitude/behaviour to their at-risk service user, the least I would expect is that you would talk about it with your colleagues and raise it in writing to the seniors of the care/support agency supplying the staff.

I remember when I was working as the head of a forensic learning disability team, we used to support service users with community activities. Occasionally, individual behaviour, described in their care plan, required us to work with people in a manner that members of the public may find difficult to understand. On the rare occasion this happened staff would hand out cards to anyone who appeared concerned with what they had witnessed. The card gave information including a phone number they could contact to talk through their concerns. For the few who phoned we gave basic information and always gave them the contact for the local social work department if they still felt concerned.

Most concerns should first be reported into the system/service where the concern has occurred. Obviously if you remain concerned or the situation is serious you should always report into the local authority safeguarding system, and if necessary other systems such as the police. All local authority websites, and doctors' surgeries, for example, contain contact details for raising safeguarding concerns.

17. Where does confidentiality/information sharing fit in?

The starting point here is that most safeguarding adult reviews, previously known as serious case reviews, identify a problem with the sharing of information, especially between agencies involved in the safeguarding process. There is a range of legislation which impacts on how we share information both internally and externally. These include: the Care Act 2014. Common law duty of confidentiality. The Human Rights Act 1998. The Data Protection Act 2018. The General Data Protection Regulation (GDPR) and the Mental Capacity Acy 2005.

What does your internal policy say about how to deal with the issue of sharing information in the situation you are presented with? How has this issue been discussed with your team? Are you confident as an employee or a manager that you would know what to share or who to talk to if the need arose? This again is part of the preparation each team should have undertaken not just for safeguarding but for general paperwork and communication.

These are questions best answered before there is a problem. Most staff I have trained state they are unsure of what the policy is in this area and therefore this area remains vulnerable were there to be a crisis.

18. What is the duty of candour?

There has always been a professional duty to be truthful and honest but as a result of the Mid Staffordshire abuse (2005–2009) and the resulting Francis Inquiry Report (published 2013) the statutory duty was introduced in November 2014 for NHS bodies such as trusts and foundation trusts in England. It was extended in April 2015 to cover all other care providers registered with the Care Quality Commission (see CQC Regulation 20).

The duty of candour is a statutory (Legal) duty to be open and honest with patients or service users or their families, when something goes wrong that appears to have caused or could lead to significant harm in the future.

If appropriate, for more details check with your professional organisation for guidance. I have included information in Appendix 2 – Useful Web Site Addresses.

19. What do I do if I feel the abuse is not deliberate?

This question almost always relates to a colleague doing something out of character from their normal. This could be, for example, speaking too abruptly when they are normally calm, or rushing a service user to do something when they normally have lots of patience. In these examples given by staff they commonly do not know what to do but are concerned by the behaviour.

Some examples are potentially more problematic, like family spending the service user's benefits in a way that supports the family and not just the service user, but that is the way they have always done it. Here staff feel there may well be no intention to cause harm. Others describe service-user-on-service-user abuse where both are at risk and there may also be capacity issues for the alleged abuser.

In all the above cases there is no option but to take it further, and we discuss how this could be done. With the first two examples it may be sufficient to raise it with the person whose behaviour is causing concern and raising it in supervision, which is recorded, with a senior.

We are not perfect, and we make mistakes sometimes depending on what is happening in our own lives. Where we are under pressure, we must improve how we pass this on to our colleagues to get support so we are less likely to transmit our feelings to our service users. Where this type of behaviour is more common, management can only support change in the staff member or family member if they know about it.

In the example with possible financial abuse this needs to be discussed with a senior/line manager to decide what to do next.

In the example of service-user-on-service-user abuse we must adopt a zero-tolerance approach, using risk assessments properly to attempt to minimise the possibility of further incidents. Learning from and debriefing after each incident are also important. Accepting levels of inappropriate behaviour is not only unacceptable but verges on organisational abuse. Capacity levels are irrelevant if you think harm may have happened.

Remember, dealing with these issues at a potentially early stage means few will need to go into referrals to the local authority but can be dealt with as management issues.

To look at one example of good practice which may already happen in other local authorities: in South Gloucestershire they encourage all person-on-person incidents be reported. Once they have reviewed the incident report and the risk assessments, they rarely progress any to enquiries, but they are all logged – as a way of building a picture of a service.

It is also important to note that whether an action, or inaction, is deliberate or not, it does not necessarily change the degree of harm.

20. What if the person allegedly being abused does not want us to raise a concern?

Where possible we should be up front with individuals we interact with by letting them know there are certain times we must report further and that we have a legal responsibility to do so. This should start with the initial paperwork we give to people we support or care for. Where necessary we should update this information on a regular basis, for example where there are known memory difficulties. While seeking consent from the individual before passing on the concern is good practice, and we should continue to seek this where possible, our legal duty is to pass on all concerns at level 3 to the local authority.

This question is usually raised by staff confused by the impact of *Making Safeguarding Personal* (see question 5). While the requirement is to involve the alleged victim of abuse, putting them at the centre of their safeguarding it is equally clear that all concerns at level 3 (question 13, step 3) must be reported both internally and to the local authority and other agencies as appropriate. We can and should ask the person what they want to happen next, but we must always raise a concern. When completing the concern paperwork, we should also pass on what the person indicated they wanted to happen (this is now a direct question on the form to be sent to the local authority). Ensuring this is passed on is essential to ensure that the reader of the concern paperwork has as much information as possible to assist them in making their decisions.

It is important to recognise why the person allegedly abused may not want to report alleged abuse, either themselves or through you.

In many cases this is dependent on the person allegedly being abused and their relationship with the alleged abuser. They may feel the abuse is more acceptable than life without the abuser; this may be especially true if they are dependent on this person and if they are family. Commonly this is seen in some areas of financial abuse and where loneliness or fear of being left unsupported without the abuser is the perception of the abused. The person may not even know they are being abused. This could be because of issues to do with capacity or their understanding of what is normal in their life. They may not want to get the staff member into trouble or fear the implications, for themselves, if they raise a concern.

As stated earlier, if we are upfront about our legal responsibilities then concerns are much more likely to be raised to us in the knowledge that we must take them further along with their wishes as to what they want to happen next.

21. What should I expect if I raise a concern?

Where you have a good manager and good practice within your team you should expect the following:

To be listened to and heard.

- To be thanked for having the confidence to raise your concern.
- To be believed in that what you are reporting you believe to be true.
- To be asked to put your concerns in writing.
- To be taken seriously.
- For your concern to be initially reviewed by your manager.
- Your concern to be passed on to the appropriate team in social services and other relevant agencies, such as the police, if required.
- To be given ongoing support during the enquiry.
- To be given reasons that satisfy you if the concern is not passed on to social services.
- To be given guidance as to what you should do next.
- To be kept informed during the process within confidentiality limits and the manager to explain some of the

constraints placed on them re disclosure organisationally and by agencies such as the police.
- To be told that your name cannot be withheld in the process from the alleged abuser where charges, either employment or criminal, are brought against the alleged abuser.
- To be debriefed, within sharing information constraints, after the enquiry is completed.
- To be reminded that you did the right thing by reporting and be thanked again.

If the above happened in every safeguarding situation there is little doubt that staff would find it easier to report. I have heard so many stories over the years where this has not happened and left the staff concerned traumatised and therefore less likely to report in the future. This is one of the reasons I developed the six steps exercise for managers (question 13), so that all staff in the team are aware of the process that comes into play from the point of raising a concern onwards.

Managers should consider compiling a checklist to ensure staff who report are not forgotten during the process but kept adequately informed and supported through what could be a traumatic situation.

Where is the incentive to report again if you feel abandoned during the process? The system includes *Making Safeguarding Personal* for the potential victims of abuse, we need to develop effective systems to protect our staff as well.

22. What can I do if I am unhappy with how a safeguarding concern is being dealt with?

This is an easy question to answer. However, it requires systems in place which give staff the confidence to use them without fear or worry about the consequences of using them. (See question 12.)

Go back to the manager and let them know you are unhappy and your reasons for your continued concern.

Ask for your concerns about the current situation to be recorded as part of your supervision, then at least there will be a record of why you were concerned. This may be enough to resolve the situation, either because the manager gave you acceptable reasons as to why decisions were not taken as you feel they should have been, or because they now took the issue further involving external agencies.

If you are genuinely worried about taking the matter further because you feel intimidated or are concerned about your employment welfare, then you should use your whistleblowing procedure. Whistleblowing procedures are a requirement for all employers as laid down in the Public Interest Disclosure Act 1998. Therefore this includes health and social care organisations. External organisations such as the police, Care Quality Commission have systems whereby anyone can contact them with concerns. The Public Interest Disclosure Act 1998 offers protection from detrimental treatment and victimisation for individual employees disclosing information on wrongdoing. There are some issues with anonymous concerns as the action taken is more likely to be diluted due to there being no one to back up the original concerns. It is always better to leave a name and contact details. However, an anonymous concern will still be taken forward to see if there is any evidence of the concern raised and, hopefully, at least logged to help build an ongoing picture.

23. What is the role of the service manager in safeguarding?

This is a key role, perhaps even *the* key role and should not be underestimated. Where there is clear evidence of good management the risk of abuse is reduced dramatically. When good managers have their finger on the pulse and are aware of what is happening within their system, communication is good, and all members of the team are more likely to feel empowered to speak freely. This in turn creates an environment where good practice is more likely to be fostered and developed.

In over 20 years training at all levels within safeguarding, I have come across many different individuals from chefs to doctors, from chief executives to porters, from nurses to support workers, from football coaches to dental hygienists. While many staff are already working to a high level of good practice it is also clear many are not as advanced as they should be. Some organisations retrain their staff every 1–3 years, so I have met many of these staff several times. While many are keen to talk about the changes since the last training, equally many appear to treat the training as mandatory box-ticking exercise and something they must endure, as opposed to want to do, and believe in. I have met staff who would not talk to their managers about concerns because they feel intimidated or believe their manager would do nothing and they would get into trouble. I have met staff who do not care and are only in the job for an income, and I have encountered different levels of understanding as to their individual role within safeguarding. It is clear, from feedback from safeguarding teams, that as a direct result of the training individuals contact the local authority in relation to a safeguarding concern that should already have been reported. In the managers training I have also encountered similar discrepancies. Most managers listen carefully and are attentive, but few take any notes. When asked at the end of their training what they may do differently many give appropriate answers, and some do not. Equally I get comments like 'I trust all my staff; abuse could not happen in my service', or 'We need to do things better but have no plan as to how to do this.' I have even heard these comments from managers whose service has been through safeguarding procedures.

I know some managers at this stage may be saying what about funding issues, salaries for staff, resources and so on? I respect that there are major issues about how we value societies most vulnerable individuals and that we should continue to campaign on these issues. However, these are red herrings when it comes to managing and developing good practice and your service. How can one service be applauded for its excellent service delivery and another similar service be in safeguarding when both are funded the same? Good practice is a state of mind as much as a physical process. Managers need to nurture and develop good practice on an ongoing basis; many of you already do.

As a professional trainer I have a responsibility to take safeguarding issues further myself if I believe it to be necessary. This is something I have had to do on a reasonably regular basis, even after all these years. Safeguarding teams in the areas where I have worked comment on how referrals increase after training sessions; this shows we still have not got clear guidelines in every team about the threshold for raising level 3 concerns.

If every manager were to implement the six steps in question 13 then we would take another important step forward.

Managers need to be trusted, respected, available, honest, consistent, supported by their seniors and juniors, approachable, good communicators, decision makers, peace makers, sensitive when required and probably a thousand other things. They need to be in control and use the systems to promote good practice. Areas such as supervision, written records, communication systems, risk assessments, training, recruitment procedures and many others are management tools which when working well automatically reduce risk. Good managers are not liked all the time because decisions they make cannot please everybody, but they should always be respected. From my own perspective respect must be earned, not just expected.

Sadly, where there is evidence of poor or weak management the risk factors increase substantially. Look at Care Quality Commission reports where excellent or good is awarded and notice their positive comments on the management of the service. Likewise, look at average and below average reports and see negative comments on the management of the system.

24. As a service manager what support should I expect from my superiors?

Much the same as your staff expect from you: to be supported, listened to, and taken seriously. (See question 21.)

Fortunately, most managers have not had to go through a serious safeguarding enquiry, especially one where it involves a member(s) of your staff team as an alleged abuser(s); you may well feel that because of you and your teams' good practice that this remains unlikely. But, like fire, which you hope will never happen, have you planned for all eventualities? Have you, during supervision with your line manager, discussed what such an enquiry may look like and what support you could reasonably be expected to receive. Surely this would be a sensible area to discuss – together you may even come up with more suggestions to make the likelihood of such an event occurring even less likely.

Again, planning is so important here. As there is an outline plan of how the process will be managed, from concern raised to enquiry completed, already laid down in the multi-agency safeguarding document, it should not be too difficult to agree an outline plan for your support during this process. To wait until it happens leaves the potential for confusion in an already traumatic situation, which should and could be avoided.

You have a responsibility to your staff, those you are paid to care/support and to yourself to work through a safeguarding enquiry professionally and competently. This is more likely with effective planning. There should be no taboos in safeguarding; everything possible should be discussed and planned for.

25. What is a section 42 enquiry (commonly known as a safeguarding enquiry)?

This relates directly to section 42 of the Care Act 2014 which states:

(1) This section applies where a local authority has reasonable cause to suspect that an adult in its area (whether or not ordinarily resident there)-
  (a) has needs for care and support (whether or not the authority is meeting any of those needs)
  (b) is experiencing, or is at risk of, abuse or neglect, and
  (c) as a result of those needs is unable to protect himself or herself against the abuse or the risk of it
(2) The local authority must make (or cause to be made) whatever enquiries it thinks necessary to enable it to decide whether any action should be taken in the adult's case (whether under this part or otherwise) and, if so, what and by whom.

(Parts 1 and 2 of Section 42 taken directly from the Care Act 2014)

As many of you will be aware there is an increasing number of concerns raised to the local authority where it is agreed that the enquiry should be carried out by those closest to the individual allegedly abused. This has been a natural evolution over several years and is recognised by the wording in the Care Act 2014 in part 2 above. Therefore, it is not uncommon for the referring organisation to work with the local authority by feeding back the result of a section 42 enquiry of their internal findings and decisions taken/to be taken.

Have you developed paperwork for your system to help you through a section 42 enquiry if it becomes your remit to carry out the enquiry and feed back to the local authority? There are many examples available on different local authority websites. I have included one of these in the useful website addresses at the end of this book. Please ensure you check to see if your local authority already has one that they require you to complete.

26. Whose policy should we follow?

There is only one policy in each local authority area. This is the multi-agency safeguarding policy, signed up to by all health and social care organisations within that area. This policy is monitored by the local safeguarding adults board and requires a consensus by the board members for amendments to the policy. The local authority safeguarding manager cannot change the multi-agency policy without consultation. They are required to submit recommendations to the local safeguarding adults board, these are then discussed, and any changes are agreed and go out for consultation to the membership of the board. Only when a consensus has been reached can any proposed changes be made. Therefore, any member of the board can recommend changes to the policy which could result in the policy being changed.

Each organisation, including social services, must also have their own internal policy which lays out how their staff should work to be compliant with the multi-agency policy.

27. What is the value of training in this area?

Back in 1999 I remember a conversation my wife, also a trainer, and I had. We were discussing the programme of rolling out safeguarding training for several local authorities and the impact it may have on our other training programmes. We were worried that when the safeguarding programmes were finished, we would have neglected our other courses to the extent it might be difficult to find enough work to keep our business viable. Twenty-one years later and safeguarding is still one of our most popular courses. I have now retired from training but will reflect on the value of training during this time and give some suggestions for the future.

The initial programmes were essential to bring all staff up to date with the new guidance coming from *No Secrets*. This started with social work staff first as they were to be the lead agency and clearly needed to develop their policies, procedures and competencies in the safeguarding process. Quickly this led onto multi-agency training. Separate training was then arranged for social workers and more senior staff in health and social care organisations. I think we naïvely thought we would carry out these training sessions and that would be that we would revert to delivering our other courses in the way we had before. We assumed that managers and organisations would take responsibility for ensuring their teams were fully informed in this area with maybe occasional updates from us if any changes happened. This, however, did not happen. We have instead been consistently providing training with staff returning about every three years for the basic awareness training. I have now trained some staff six or seven times in the raising-concerns course.

The most successful courses I have run in safeguarding have been where a whole team has trained together. In those situations, you can concentrate on one team, one system and develop a meaningful action plan. Concentration levels are higher as areas being discussed affect all the participants involved.

The basic problem with multi-agency training, on an ongoing basis, in safeguarding is a lack of ownership. There may be up ten organisations represented in a group of eighteen participants. The participants may range from catering, finance, nursing, social worker, support worker to chief executive, doctor, physiotherapist. Meeting such diverse needs can be a real challenge, and not only for the trainer. More importantly this type of training expects those motivated by the training to go back and stimulate change within their team. While this may be a viable option for senior staff within the team it is much more difficult for staff who may feel powerless within their team. It certainly does not help when at least one person per course asks if they are on this session as they were only told where and when the training was taking place, not why they were there. This surely shows a lack of management commitment.

There is a need for a multitude of training options to be available to individual and teams. These include whole team training, on-the-job training, e-learning and multi-agency training. Using only one of these methods is unlikely to be successful. Good managers already know this and use this variety of methods to get the best out of their staff. They also accept the different ways their staff learn. Some staff are very practical, dyslexic, scared by what they perceive as academia and learn best by on-the-job training, while they may learn little by classroom training. Others may excel at conversation and learn better in a group setting.

Training should not be seen as an add-on to satisfy the needs of audit checks. Training should be a core essential if we are truly to value our staff and service. Therefore, there needs to be discussion before the training as to why staff are going on a particular course and agreed expectations. This then needs to be followed up post training to find out how the training has influenced the trainee and any changes in practice noted. This should also help to raise issues with poor training from individual trainers. Otherwise, a valuable and at times costly resource may be wasted.

Remember, if you are reporting at level 3, then if you are unhappy with current outcomes, you have the right and legal responsibility to take it further yourself to, for example, the local authority safeguarding team, police or Care Quality Commission, if registered.

To be able to do any of the above more easily you need to be working in a system that respects staff and has robust systems that allow staff to feel comfortable to take this concern further. Unfortunately, I have come across too many staff who feel that after reporting further their job is done, and to question decisions would be putting their head above the parapet and leave themselves vulnerable.

This is another area where managers need to review how their staff should question decisions and how this would work in their team, which again brings us back to the need for planning and minimising potential problems during this process.

If you are working in a multi-agency setting where there are a group of professionals from different organisations involved, for example, care and support staff, community nurses, domiciliary care staff, day care staff and perhaps other visiting professionals, remember the escalation policy (within your safeguarding policy).

28. What is the role of the Care Quality Commission?

The Care Quality Commission are the independent regulator of health and social care in England. Services regulated by the Care Quality Commission are as follows:

- Care homes.
- Hospitals.
- Services in your home.
- Doctors/GPS.
- Dentists.
- Clinics.
- Community services.
- Mental health services.

Within their fundamental standards are safety, safeguarding from abuse and duty of candour. These are standards set, below which your care must never fall. To see all the fundamental standards Appendix 2 has the website for the Care Quality Commission.

Their purpose is to make sure health and social care services provide people with safe, effective, compassionate, high quality care and encourage care services to improve.

Their roles are to register care providers, monitor, inspect and rate services, take action to protect people who use services and to speak with an independent voice, publishing their views on major quality issues in health and social care.

Anyone who sees the role of the Care Quality Commission as the sole upholders of good practice in every regulated service is sadly deluded. Their role is vital and important, but they cannot be everywhere all the time. They rely on us, all of us, from staff, relatives to concerned members of the public, to bring to their attention concerns we may have about safeguarding issues. Remember, safeguarding is everyone's business.

The Care Quality Commission are promoters and sharers of good practice, they cannot be held fully responsible for missing individual safeguarding situations, especially where staff and others have concerns but have not shared them.

From a safeguarding perspective, remember your legal requirements, especially under Regulation 13: Safeguarding service users from abuse and improper treatment. (Health and Social Care Act 2008 (Regulated Activities) Regulations 2014 and Regulation 20 Duty of Candour.)

29. What is the difference between individual and organisational abuse?

Individual abuse usually refers to abuse towards one person at risk by an individual or individuals.

Cases reported to the local authority can range from a single contact where it is accepted by all parties that the risk has either been eliminated or is being effectively managed with the case closed at this stage.

Examples here could include:

- A medication error where no harm is caused to the individual and a new procedure for administration of medications has been written which makes such errors much less likely.
- A resident has had several falls, including one where she broke her wrist. On reporting to the local authority due to the harm caused it is found that the home has all sensible precautions in place, such as aids and adaptations, falls professionals from the local health service involved, records clear and in place, updated care plan information about steps to make falls less likely.

Most cases reported in individual abuse are dealt with quickly by the gathering of information and agencies working with the local authority to manage the risk more effectively. Strategy discussions, usually by phone, are more common than strategy meetings, gathering people round a table, in individual abuse. In these cases, small numbers of staff are normally involved in strategy discussions/meetings.

Other cases reported into safeguarding may be protracted and involve a multi-agency approach with meetings/discussions over a longer period. This will include cases where the police view the report as criminal and start their procedures. Cases involving domestic abuse, theft, physical assault and sexual abuse are the most common in this area.

The local authority has the sole ability to decide when a safeguarding case is closed, conferred on them by the Care Act 2014. There is a clear procedure to be followed and they can close a case at any point in the procedure when they are satisfied the risk has been eliminated or is being professionally managed. Other professionals can challenge decisions made by using the escalation policy.

Organisational abuse usually refers to a services practice that is abusive towards individuals at risk within that service, the systems employed by the organisation, or part of the organisation, may be abusive towards multiple individuals at risk within that service. Although not exclusively, most organisational abuse cases originate from residential and hospital areas where groups of individuals at risk are cared for or supported. This can range from a small group home to a large nursing home, hospital or day service.

Cases raised with or by the local authority may include:

- An organisation that has not updated their practices for many years and are now working in a way that may be abusive.
- Restrictive practices such as routines established for staff convenience but not meeting the individual needs of service users.
- A group of staff behaving in an unacceptable manner, e.g., levels of control, aggression (verbal or physical) towards service users.
- Not learning from previous safeguarding cases, e.g., medication errors, falls.
- Not meeting training requirements including mandatory and professional development requirements for safe practice.
- Not using required equipment or aids or not using them as specified in the care plan.

Cases may come to the attention of the local authority from many sources. These may include visiting professionals, individuals receiving the service, from staff within the team, relatives, issues identified by the Care Quality Commission during inspections, issues raised by other local authority staff where they have individual(s) placed out of their own authority area and are carrying out reviews, concerned members of the public.

Sometimes cases come to the attention of the local authority because, on checking, no safeguarding/deprivation of liberty referrals have been received and on visiting the service safeguarding staff identify concerns themselves.

Often the safeguarding referral is in relation to one service user, but then further referrals come in affecting other service users in the same service.

30. How are organisational abuse enquiries carried out?

The biggest difference between individual abuse and organisational abuse is that enquiries tend to be large-scale enquiries as a rule. The number of people involved therefore also tends to be much larger, making meetings more intimidating to those present. They also tend to be longer meetings and remain in safeguarding for a longer period as the need to sort systems and procedures often is a drawn-out process to ensure changes are bedded in.

People who could be present at an organisational abuse safeguarding meeting may include:

- Representatives of the organisation undergoing safeguarding enquiry.
- Safeguarding team members from the local authority.
- Representatives from other local authorities who have individuals placed in the affected service.
- Care Quality Commission.
- Police.
- Representatives of those allegedly abused.
- Other health and social care professionals dependant on the case e.g., GP, community psychiatric nurse, occupational therapist, pharmacist.
- Legal representatives from the local authority.

- Media representatives from the local authority.
- Contracts representatives from the local authority.
- Minute taker.

Meetings are the norm in these enquiries as opposed to phone discussions. This is to allow for sharing information and planning and monitoring changes required. There may be anything from 10–50 individuals present at these meetings, depending on the scale of the enquiry. These meetings will be chaired by the local authority adult safeguarding team staff. Once introductions have been made and confidentiality agreements are in place the meeting can begin.

The aim of the initial meeting is to lay out the concerns being raised. This means giving time to each person present to raise their concerns. For the organisation under safeguarding procedures this is a difficult meeting, as their service is the one being discussed. Normally, once all the concerns have been raised then the organisation under safeguarding procedures replies to these concerns. It is important that the organisation in safeguarding procedures ensures that their staff present have the authority to make decisions and that there is more than one present to offer support and advice.

The purpose of this meeting is to prepare an initial action plan for resolving the issues raised, agreeing support for the organisation and service users and setting timescales for improvements and who will be responsible for feeding back on each of the areas of improvement required.

Subsequent meetings are to monitor and if appropriate to amend the action plan, monitor the timescales and ensure the changes being implemented are sustainable and working.

While most of the changes recommended are the responsibility of the organisation under review to complete, additional support from other stakeholders such as health and social care professionals is agreed at the initial and subsequent meetings.

An additional complication presents itself where police believe criminal activity may have taken place and start their procedures

This causes obvious time delays to the safeguarding process, and increased pressure within an already complicated situation.

Having trained managers from organisations who have been through an organisational abuse enquiry and moved their service forward in a positive manner, their comments are worth recording. Most say the initial meeting was very difficult and uncomfortable but agreed that the support and timescales and targets set were valuable to moving their service forward. Most also thanked the safeguarding staff at the end of the process and accepted their service was much improved from the service that entered safeguarding procedures.

In extreme cases where the changes are either not working or being actively worked against by the organisation under safeguarding procedures, the Care Quality Commission has the power to close the service.

31. How are staff protected by safeguarding?

There are two quite different answers to this question, depending on how the question is asked.

Firstly, as a direct question, the answer is that if all participants are following set policies and procedures to a high level of good practice then the likelihood of safeguarding incidents at all three levels are greatly reduced. Therefore, we give ourselves a level of protection from having to be involved in reacting to abuse, in the first place, by our own high levels of good practice. (There is also direct legislation to protect staff, for example the Health and Safety Act 1974 requires risk assessments to be undertaken in relation to both quantifying the risk and giving guidance as to how staff should work with that risk in the safest manner for both the individual and themselves).

Secondly, when this question is raised, normally, what is being asked is how does safeguarding protect staff where they are being abused by, for example, a person at risk they are supporting/caring for, or by partners or family members. The answer is simple, safeguarding procedures are there to protect the people we support, not the staff. However, as already stated, if we safeguard all properly, we reduce the likelihood of staff being at risk.

Because this area is raised by someone in almost every raising-concerns group I want to delve further. Many staff feel we have policies to protect those we support but have nothing similar for staff, and therefore feel unprotected. We discuss which groups they are talking about who may cause them to feel this way. The main groups mentioned include people with:

- Dementia.
- Behaviour that challenges us to understand it.
- Addictions.
- Mental health.
- Waiting in waiting rooms, e.g., outpatients.
- Coercive partners during home visits.

We then discuss what types of behaviour they have or worry about experiencing. This includes anything from being sworn at, assaulted (from hair-pulling to being punched), intimidation, to being shouted at. I ask then how many of them have it in their job description that it is acceptable to be sworn at or assaulted. Obviously, they all agree they do not have this in their job description. We then move onto zero tolerance for unacceptable behaviour and how this should be discussed, risk-assessed and worked through within their systems aimed at protecting staff. We identify policies from supervision, recording, de-briefing and accident reporting.

The fact that there is a need to do this with almost every group indicates to me that this is an area of concern where many staff do not feel protected. I have too frequently had staff say to me, for example, 'I work with people with dementia/behaviour that challenges us/post-operative anaesthesia and being hit is just part of the job.' More worrying, some managers support this belief. It is not part of the job, and while even one member of staff believes this to be true, there is a problem.

The fact is that every organisation is obliged to have clear and accessible policies and procedures covering issues from preventing harassment and bullying to preventing violence and aggression against staff and other forms of unacceptable behaviours. Who in your organisation is reviewing the use and impact of these policies? I see the problem not being with the policies and procedures but with individual staff not using these policies when they should. More consideration should be given to why they are not confident enough to use them effectively. Failure to do this already results in some staff feeling undervalued within their service and less likely to take concerns further.

32. What is the impact of abuse?

During training sessions, we look at this from a group-by-group perspective and the participants quickly realise that the same points are raised by each group, therefore, to avoid repetition I will give an overview.

The impact of abuse can range from minimal, i.e., where a medication error has occurred and no apparent harm was caused to the individual, to severe, i.e., financial abuse where police prosecutions and convictions have occurred.

The impact of abuse can be felt by a variety of individuals or groups dependant on the individual situation, but can include:

- The victim of abuse.
- The staff team especially heightened where the alleged perpetrator is a colleague.
- Family members and friends.
- Other members of the external multi-professional team.

Impacts of abuse most often expressed are:

- Guilt/Could I have done more/How did I not know?
- Lack of trust.

- Disbelief that this has happened, or that a colleague was responsible.
- Helplessness.
- Anger.
- Depression.
- Need for justice.
- Need for information.

Has your team discussed the above list and the impact it may have on you, and others, if you were to be involved in a safeguarding case? Have you discussed that these feelings are perfectly normal, and have you agreed how you would professionally work through the situation? Can you imagine trying to work through a safeguarding case, with the above symptoms present, affecting different groups, without any planning and preparation already in place to guide your staff on how to remain professional and competent in the carrying out of their regular duties?

Appendix 1 Early Indicators of Concern in Care Services (Organisational Abuse)

Taken from South Gloucestershire Safeguarding Adults Board Organisational Abuse Procedures 2021

Checklist

It is important to note that this is not a definitive checklist. Other indicators may be identified that do not appear on this list.

1. Concerns about management and leadership:

The manager of the service:

- The manager leaves suddenly and unexpectedly.
- The service has not had a registered manager in post over an extended period.
- Arrangements to cover the service while the manager is away not working well.
- The manager is new and does not appear to understand what the service is set up to do.
- A responsible manager is not apparent or available within the service and has little involvement with the adults.
- The manager leaves staff to get on with things with little active guidance or modelling of good practice.
- The manager is very controlling.

Management culture:

- The service is not being managed in a planned way, but reacts to problems and crises.
- The service does not respond appropriately when a serious incident has taken place.
- The service fails to learn from previous incidents and does

not appear to be taking steps to reduce the risk of a similar incident happening again.
- Policies, procedures and practice guidance are absent or inadequate.

The management team:

- Senior staff have been in post a long time and have a high level of authority and entrenched views.
- There is a high turnover of managers.
- The service is experiencing difficulty in recruiting and appointing managers.
- There is a lack of leadership by managers, for example managers do not make decisions and set priorities.
- Managers appear unaware of serious problems in the service.
- Managers do not appear to be attending to risk assessments or are not ensuring that risk assessments have been carried out properly.
- Managers do not appear to have ensured that staff have information about individual adults' needs and potential risks to adults.
- Managers appear unable to ensure that actions agreed at reviews and other meetings are followed through.
- There is a lack of effective monitoring by senior staff – including support to night staff and checks on them.
- The managers know what outcomes should be delivered for adults, but appear unable to organise the service to deliver these outcomes, i.e. they appear unable to 'make it happen'.

Staffing:

- Staff who raise issues are not listened to.
- Staff are not being deployed effectively to meet the needs of adults.

- There is a high turnover of staff.
- Staff are working long hours.
- Staff are working when they are ill.
- There is poor staff morale.
- Recruitment processes are inadequate.
- The service employs high numbers of family/friends.
- There is a failure to identify concerning behaviour by staff, e.g. stressed staff behaving unusually, growth of cliques, failure to work to best practice, cutting corners.
- The managers have low expectations of the staff.
- Staff have poor pay and conditions of employment.

2. Concerns about staff skills, knowledge and practice:

Supervision and training:

- Staff receive little/no supervision, appraisals or opportunities for development.
- Induction processes are inadequate.
- Poor quality or no training is provided.
- Staff appear to lack the information, knowledge and skills needed to support the people the service is set up to support.
- Staff lack training in how to use equipment.

Recording:

- Record keeping by staff is poor.
- Staff do not appear to see keeping records as important.
- Risk assessments are not completed or are of poor quality. For example, they lack details or do not identify significant risks.
- Incident reports are not being completed.
- Records are value laden and judgemental.

Mental capacity and DOLS:

- There is non-adherence to the principles of the Mental Capacity Act.
- There is a lack of understanding of DOLS.
- DOLS referrals are not being made, resulting in people being unlawfully deprived of their liberty.

Interactions with adults:

- Staff appear challenged by some adults' behaviours and do not manage these in a safe, professional or dignified way.
- Staff perceive the behaviours of adults as a problem – and blame the adults.
- Staff blame adults' medical condition for all their difficulties, needs and behaviours; other explanations do not appear to be considered.
- Adults are punished for behaviours seen to be inappropriate.
- Staff treat adults roughly or forcefully.
- Staff ignore adults.
- Staff are impatient with adults.
- Staff talk to adults in ways which are derogatory/not complimentary.
- Staff shout or swear at adults.
- Staff do not alter their communication style to meet individual needs. For example, they speak to people as if they are children, they 'jolly people along'.
- Staff use negative or judgemental language when talking about adults.
- Staff do not see adults as individuals and do not appear aware of their life history.
- Staff do not ensure privacy for people when providing personal care.
- Staff tell adults to use their incontinence pads rather than assist them to use the toilet.

Culture:

- There is a particular group of staff who strongly influence how things happen in the home.
- Staff informally complain about the managers to visiting professionals.
- Staff appear to lack interest and commitment.
- Staff appear to lack concern for the adults.
- Staff appear unable to relate to a particular adult.
- Staff are complacent about the quality of care they provide and appear defensive when challenged.

3. Concerns about adults' behaviours and wellbeing:

Individual adults:

- Show signs of injury due to lack of care or attention (e.g., as a result of not using wheelchairs carefully or properly, or the development of pressure injuries due to lack of or inappropriate use of pressure relieving equipment).
- Appear frightened or show signs of fear.
- Behaviours or appearances have changed, for example they have become unkempt or are no longer taking pride or interest in their appearance.
- Moods or psychological presentation have changed.
- Behaviour is different with certain members of staff/when certain members of staff are away.
- Engage in inappropriate sexualised behaviours.
- Do not progress as would be expected.
- Experience sensory deprivation – e.g., going without spectacles or hearing aids.
- Experience restricted mobility by being denied access to mobility aids.
- Experience restricted access to toilet/bathing facilities.
- Lack personal clothing and/or possessions.

General service concerns:

- The overall atmosphere is flat, gloomy or miserable.
- There is a high number of low-level incidents such as medication errors or falls.
- There is a high number of incidents between adults.
- There are a high number of upheld complaints about the service.
- There is evidence of inappropriate restraint methods or misused restraint, including the inappropriate use of medication.
- The care regime exhibits lack of choice, flexibility and control.
- The care regime appears impersonal and lacks respect for individual's privacy and dignity.

4. Concerns about the service resisting the involvement of external people and isolating individuals:

Information sharing:

- The service has few visitors/minimal outside contacts.
- The service does not report safeguarding concerns.
- The service does not communicate with or report concerns to external practitioners and agencies.
- The service does not liaise with families and ignores their offers of help and support.
- Managers and/or staff do not respond to advice or guidance from practitioners and families who visit the service.
- Managers do not appear to provide staff with information about adults from meetings with external people, for example reviews.
- Staff or managers appear defensive or hostile and concerned to avoid blame when questions or problems are raised by external practitioners or families.

- Managers or staff give inconsistent responses or accounts of situations.

Staff:

- Staff work alone on a one-to-one basis with adults.
- Staff work in silos e.g., night staff who never work days.
- Staff are hostile towards or ignore practitioners and families who visit the service.

Adults:

- There are adults who have little contact with people from outside the service.
- There are adults who are not receiving active monitoring or reviews (e.g., people who are self-funding).
- Adults are kept isolated in their rooms and are unable to move to other parts of the building or outside independently ('enforced isolation').
- Adults have restricted access to visitors or phone calls.
- Adults have restricted access to health or social care services.

5. Concerns about the way services are planned and delivered:

The nature of the service:

- The service does not have a clear philosophy/purpose.
- The service does not appear able to deliver the service or support it is commissioned to provide. For example, it is unable to deliver effective support to people with distressed or aggressive behaviour..
- Decisions about what service is commissioned for an individual are influenced by a lack of suitable alternatives.
- The service is accepting adults whose needs and/or

behaviours are different to those of the adults previously or usually accepted.
- The service is accepting adults whose needs they appear unable to meet.
- Adults' needs as identified in assessments, care plans or risk assessments are not being met. For example, adults are not being supported to attend specific activities or provided with specific support to enable them to remain safe.

Person-centred care:

- Staff are task focused and not providing person-centred care.
- Adults are treated en-mass.
- The service follows strict, regimented routines – for mealtimes, bedtimes, etc.
- Adults lack choice about food and drink, dress, possessions, activities and where they want to spend their time.
- Members of staff are controlling of adults.
- There are misunderstandings about confidentiality.

Resources:

- There is a failure to provide and/or maintain correct moving and handling and other equipment such as pressure relieving mattresses.
- The service is under resourced – whether staff, equipment or provisions.
- There appear to be insufficient staff to support adults appropriately.

Audits:

- There is a lack of audits of practice and process.
- There is a failure to follow up on issues raised by audits.
- There is a failure to monitor the use of call bells including checking they have not been disabled – especially at night.

6. Concerns about the quality of basic care and the environment:

Person-centred care:

- There is a lack of privacy, dignity and respect for people as individuals.
- There is a lack of provision for dress, diet or religious observance in accordance with adults' individual beliefs or cultural backgrounds.
- Adults do not have as much money as would be expected.
- Adults lack basic things such as clothes, toiletries.
- Support for adults to maintain personal hygiene and cleanliness is poor and they appear unkempt.
- Adults are not getting the support they need with eating and drinking, or are not getting enough to eat or drink.
- There is poor or inadequate support for adults who have health problems or who need medical attention.
- Staff are not checking that people are safe and well.
- There are a lack of activities or social opportunities for adults.
- There is a lack of care for adults' property and clothing.

Resources:

- There appear to be insufficient staff to meet adults' needs.
- The service does not have the equipment needed to support adults and keep them safe.
- Equipment or furniture is broken.

- Equipment is not being used or is not being used safely and correctly.

Environment:

- The service is not providing a safe environment.
- The environment is dirty and shows signs of poor hygiene.
- The quality of the environment has deteriorated noticeably.

Appendix 2 Useful Websites

www.gov.uk   Care Act 2014
            Care Act factsheets

www.scie.org.uk Making Safeguarding Personal and many other headings relevant to adult safeguarding.

www.ihm.org.uk / duty-of-candour-at-a-glance

www.cqc.org.uk

www.nhs.uk >Documents PDF Quick guide: Sharing patient information.

www.informationsharing.org.uk

Your local authority website will contain useful information around various aspects of adult safeguarding relevant to your local area.

Sharing Good Practice Series

Down Syndrome and Dementia – 2020
Safeguarding Adults – 2021

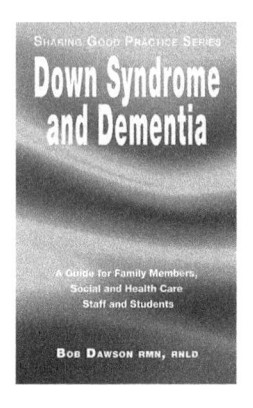

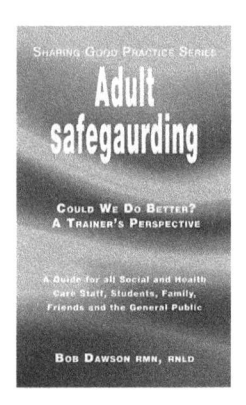

Reviews for Down Syndrome and Dementia

Jan 2021 – 'It's a really great read.' Kelly Brien, Service Manager, Ambito (Salutem Healthcare)

Jan 2021 – 'The guide was so enlightening, and I look forward to developing some resources for the people I work with to support their practice. Thank you again for producing something so clear and relevant.' Tracey Barnes RNLD

'This book is an easy read. It addresses lots of issues that worry and concern people supporting and caring for people with Down Syndrome and Dementia. This is clearly based on the author's many years of practice, but also on training sessions, which have highlighted the areas of concern. The result is a book written with the author's voice and a light touch. It is accessible, well informed, and full of important messages about good practice in the support of people with learning disabilities who are living with dementia.' Diana Kerr Training Consultant and Author